ENDOMETRIOSIS AND FERTILITY:

Treatment Options and Considerations

By

MARTIN S. COLLINS

LEGAL NOTICE

You are encouraged to print this book for easy reading.

TABLE OF CONTENTS

INTRODUCTION

Endometriosis is a condition where tissue similar to the lining of the uterus grows outside of the uterus, causing pain and discomfort. While endometriosis affects an estimated 10% of reproductive-aged women, it is often associated with fertility problems. Endometriosis can interfere with ovulation, damage the fallopian tubes, and cause inflammation that can prevent the implantation of a fertilized egg.

For women with endometriosis who are trying to conceive, there is a range of treatment options and considerations to be aware of. In some cases, lifestyle changes such as a healthy diet and regular exercise can help to manage symptoms and improve fertility. In other cases, medications such as hormone therapies may be used to reduce inflammation and promote ovulation. Surgery to remove endometriosis tissue or to repair any damage to the reproductive organs may also be necessary.

It's important for women with endometriosis who are trying to conceive to work closely with their healthcare providers to develop a personalized treatment plan that takes into account their individual needs and goals. By addressing endometriosis symptoms and managing any related fertility issues, women with endometriosis can improve their chances of conceiving and carrying out a healthy pregnancy.

Endometriosis can have a significant impact on fertility and can make it more difficult for women to conceive. This is because endometriosis can cause a range of issues that can interfere with the normal reproductive process. For example, endometriosis can cause the formation of adhesions, or scar tissue, in the pelvis, which can block the fallopian tubes and prevent the egg and sperm from meeting. Additionally, endometriosis can cause inflammation and scarring in the uterus, making it more difficult for a fertilized egg to implant and grow.

There are several treatment options available to help women with endometriosis who are trying to conceive.

One common approach is to use medications to regulate hormones and reduce inflammation. Hormonal treatments such as birth control pills, gonadotropin-releasing hormone (GnRH) agonists, and progestins can help to reduce the growth of endometriosis tissue and relieve symptoms such as pain and heavy bleeding. These medications can also help to promote ovulation and improve fertility.

Surgery may also be an option for women with endometriosis who are trying to conceive. Laparoscopic surgery, which involves using a thin, flexible instrument to remove endometriosis tissue or repair any damage to the reproductive organs, can help to improve fertility and increase the chances of conception. In some cases, more extensive surgery such as a hysterectomy may be necessary.

CHAPTER ONE

UNDERSTANDING ENDOMETRIOSIS AND ITS IMPACT ON FERTILITY

Endometriosis is a medical condition in which the tissue that lines the inside of the uterus (called the endometrium) grows outside of it. This tissue can grow on the ovaries, fallopian tubes, bladder, and other organs in the pelvis. This can cause severe pain during periods, pain during sex, and fertility problems.

The exact cause of endometriosis is unknown, but it is believed to be related to hormonal imbalances and genetic factors. The condition affects about 10% of women of reproductive age, and it can be difficult to diagnose because its symptoms can vary greatly and be similar to other conditions.

Endometriosis can have a significant impact on fertility. It can cause scarring and adhesions in the pelvis, which can make it difficult for the ovaries and fallopian tubes to function properly. This can lead to infertility or an increased risk of miscarriage. Additionally, the inflammation caused by endometriosis can harm the eggs and sperm, making conception more difficult.

Treatment for endometriosis depends on the severity of the condition and the patient's goals for fertility. Mild cases may be managed with pain medication and hormonal treatments that can suppress the growth of the tissue. More severe cases may require surgery to remove the tissue and repair any damage to the reproductive organs.

In some cases, fertility treatments such as in vitro fertilization (IVF) may be necessary to help women with endometriosis conceive. IVF involves retrieving eggs from the ovaries, fertilizing them with sperm in a laboratory, and then transferring the resulting embryos into the uterus.

It is important for women who are experiencing symptoms of endometriosis or who are having difficulty getting pregnant to speak with their healthcare provider. Early diagnosis and treatment can help to manage symptoms and increase the chances of a successful pregnancy.

Medical Treatments for Endometriosis and Effects on Fertility

Medical treatments for endometriosis aim to relieve symptoms, slow the growth of endometrial tissue, and prevent the formation of new lesions. These treatments can include:

1. Hormonal Therapy: Hormonal therapy is often used as a first-line treatment for endometriosis. It works by suppressing the production of estrogen, which is known to stimulate the growth of endometrial tissue. Hormonal therapies may include birth control pills, progestins, GnRH agonists, or danazol.

2. Nonsteroidal Anti-inflammatory Drugs (NSAIDs): NSAIDs such as ibuprofen and naproxen can be effective in reducing the pain associated with endometriosis.

3. Surgery: Surgery may be necessary in cases of severe endometriosis or when fertility is a

concern. Surgery can involve removing endometrial tissue, scar tissue, and adhesions. It can also involve removing or repairing any damaged reproductive organs.

The effects of medical treatments for endometriosis on fertility can vary. Hormonal therapies can temporarily halt ovulation, which can make it more difficult to conceive. However, once the therapy is stopped, ovulation typically resumes. Additionally, hormonal therapies can be used in conjunction with fertility treatments such as intrauterine insemination (IUI) or in vitro fertilization (IVF).

Surgery for endometriosis can improve fertility in some cases by removing scar tissue and adhesions that can interfere with ovulation and fertilization. However, surgery is not always a guarantee of improved fertility, and the extent of any fertility improvement will depend on the severity of the endometriosis and any damage that has occurred to the reproductive organs.

In summary, medical treatments for endometriosis can be effective in managing symptoms and slowing the growth of endometrial tissue. However, the effects of these treatments on fertility can vary, and women with endometriosis who are trying to conceive should work closely with their healthcare provider to develop a treatment plan that is tailored to their individual needs and goals.

CHAPTER TWO

SURGICAL INTERVENTIONS FOR ENDOMETRIOSIS: BENEFITS AND RISKS FOR FERTILITY

Surgical intervention for endometriosis involves the removal of endometrial tissue, scar tissue, and adhesions that can cause pain and infertility. There are several types of surgical interventions for endometriosis, including laparoscopy, laparotomy, and robotic-assisted laparoscopic surgery.

Laparoscopy is the most common surgical procedure for endometriosis. It is a minimally invasive procedure in which a small incision is made in the abdomen and a laparoscope (a thin tube with a camera) is inserted to view the inside of the abdomen. Small instruments are used to remove endometrial tissue and any adhesions.

Laparotomy is a more invasive surgery that involves making a larger incision in the abdomen. This type of surgery may be necessary for more severe cases of endometriosis or when there is significant scarring and adhesions.

Robotic-assisted laparoscopic surgery is a newer technique that uses a robotic arm to control the laparoscope and instruments. This type of surgery can be more precise and less invasive than traditional laparoscopic surgery.

Benefits of surgical intervention for endometriosis include:

1. Reduction of pain: Surgery can remove endometrial tissue and scar tissue, which can reduce pain associated with endometriosis.
2. Improved fertility: Surgery can remove adhesions and scar tissue, which can improve fertility by improving the function of the ovaries and fallopian tubes.
3. Diagnosis: Surgery can be used to confirm a diagnosis of endometriosis and identify the extent and severity of the disease.

Risks of surgical intervention for endometriosis include:

1. Complications from surgery: Like any surgery, there are risks of bleeding, infection, and damage to surrounding organs.
2. Recurrence of endometriosis: Endometriosis can recur after surgery, especially if all of the endometrial tissue is not removed.
3. Scarring: Surgery can cause additional scarring, which can lead to further fertility problems.

Surgical intervention for endometriosis can be an effective treatment option for reducing pain and improving fertility. However, it is important to carefully weigh the benefits and risks of surgery and to work with a skilled surgeon who has experience in treating endometriosis. Women with endometriosis who are considering surgery should discuss their options with their healthcare provider to determine the best course of treatment for their individual needs and goals.

Fertility Preservation Options for Women with Endometriosis

Endometriosis can have a significant impact on fertility, and women with the condition who wish to preserve their fertility have several options. Fertility preservation involves preserving eggs or embryos so that they can be used in the future when a woman is ready to conceive.

1. Egg Freezing: Egg freezing, also known as oocyte cryopreservation, involves retrieving a woman's eggs and freezing them for later use. This is typically done through a process called in vitro fertilization (IVF), in which the eggs are retrieved from the ovaries and frozen immediately. Egg freezing can be a good option for women with endometriosis who may need to undergo surgery or hormonal treatments that could potentially damage their ovaries and diminish their ovarian reserve.

2. Embryo Freezing: Embryo freezing involves fertilizing a woman's eggs with sperm in a laboratory to create embryos, which are then

frozen for later use. This option is typically used for women who have a partner and who are planning to undergo IVF treatment.

3. Ovarian Tissue Freezing: Ovarian tissue freezing involves removing a small piece of a woman's ovary and freezing it for later use. This option is still considered experimental, and it is typically only recommended for women who are facing certain medical treatments that could damage their ovaries, such as chemotherapy or radiation therapy.

Fertility preservation options can be costly, and they may not be covered by insurance. Women with endometriosis who are interested in preserving their fertility should discuss their options with their healthcare provider and a fertility specialist to determine the best course of action for their individual needs and goals.

CHAPTER THREE

PSYCHOLOGICAL SUPPORT FOR WOMEN WITH ENDOMETRIOSIS AND FERTILITY CONCERNS

Endometriosis is a painful and often debilitating condition where tissue similar to the lining of the uterus grows outside of the uterus. This condition can have a significant impact on a woman's physical and emotional health, including fertility concerns. Psychological support can play an important role in helping women with endometriosis cope with their symptoms and address fertility concerns.

Here are some ways psychological support can be beneficial for women with endometriosis and fertility concerns:

1. Coping with pain and symptoms: Chronic pain and other symptoms associated with endometriosis can be difficult to manage and can significantly impact a woman's quality of life. Psychological support can help women

learn coping strategies to manage their pain and symptoms and improve their overall well-being.

2. Managing stress and anxiety: Endometriosis and fertility concerns can be stressful and cause anxiety. Psychological support can help women manage stress and anxiety and reduce the impact of these emotions on their physical health.

3. Addressing fertility concerns: Endometriosis can affect a woman's fertility, which can be a significant concern for many women. Psychological support can help women explore their options for fertility treatment, manage the emotional stress of infertility, and make informed decisions about their reproductive health.

4. Improving communication with healthcare providers: Women with endometriosis and fertility concerns may have difficulty communicating with their healthcare providers. Psychological support can help women develop

communication skills to effectively express their concerns and questions to their providers.

5. Providing a supportive environment: Endometriosis and fertility concerns can be isolating and make women feel alone. Psychological support can provide a supportive environment where women can connect with others who are experiencing similar challenges and receive encouragement and support.

Overall, psychological support can play an important role in helping women with endometriosis and fertility concerns cope with their symptoms, manage their emotions, and improve their overall well-being. Women need to seek out qualified mental health professionals with experience in working with women with endometriosis and fertility concerns to receive the most appropriate and effective support.

Alternative and Complementary Therapies for Endometriosis and Fertility

Alternative and complementary therapies are often sought out by women with endometriosis and fertility concerns as a way to manage symptoms and improve overall well-being. While these therapies may not cure endometriosis or guarantee pregnancy, they can be used in conjunction with traditional medical treatments to enhance overall health and improve quality of life. Here are some alternative and complementary therapies that may be beneficial for women with endometriosis and fertility concerns:

1. Acupuncture: Acupuncture is a form of traditional Chinese medicine that involves inserting thin needles into specific points of the body. Acupuncture has been shown to help reduce pain and inflammation associated with endometriosis, as well as improve fertility by promoting blood flow to the reproductive organs.

2. Herbal medicine: Some herbs may be beneficial for managing endometriosis symptoms and improving fertility. Examples include turmeric, ginger, and chaste berry. However, it's important to note that herbal remedies can have side effects and may interact with other

medications. It's essential to speak with a qualified herbalist or healthcare provider before using herbal remedies.

3. Mind-body techniques: Mind-body techniques such as meditation, yoga, and tai chi can help reduce stress and promote relaxation, which may help manage endometriosis symptoms and improve overall well-being.

4. Nutrition and supplements: A healthy diet and certain supplements may be beneficial for managing endometriosis symptoms and improving fertility. Examples include omega-3 fatty acids, vitamin D, and magnesium.

5. Manual therapy: Manual therapy such as osteopathy or chiropractic care can help alleviate pain and improve mobility associated with endometriosis.

Alternative and complementary therapies should not be used as a substitute for medical treatment. Women with endometriosis and fertility concerns should work with their healthcare provider to develop a comprehensive treatment plan that includes both traditional medical treatments and alternative and complementary therapies. It's essential to seek out qualified practitioners and to inform healthcare providers of any alternative or complementary therapies being used.

CHAPTER FOUR

LIFESTYLE MODIFICATIONS TO IMPROVE FERTILITY OUTCOMES IN ENDOMETRIOSIS

Making lifestyle modifications can be an effective way to improve fertility outcomes in women with endometriosis. Here are some lifestyle modifications that may be beneficial:

1. Diet and Nutrition: Eating a healthy and balanced diet can improve fertility outcomes for women with endometriosis. A diet rich in antioxidants, vitamins, and minerals, such as vitamin C, vitamin E, and folic acid, can help reduce inflammation and oxidative stress in the body. It is also important to avoid foods that may trigger inflammation, such as processed foods, refined carbohydrates, and sugar.

2. Regular Exercise: Regular exercise has been shown to improve fertility outcomes in women with endometriosis. Exercise can help reduce stress and inflammation, which can improve overall health and fertility. It is important to choose a type of exercise that is low impact and does not exacerbate endometriosis symptoms.

3. Stress Management: Chronic stress can negatively impact fertility outcomes for women with endometriosis. Engaging in stress-reducing activities, such as yoga, meditation, and mindfulness, can help reduce stress and improve fertility outcomes.

4. Sleep: Getting enough sleep is important for overall health and fertility. Women with endometriosis should aim to get 7-8 hours of sleep each night to support hormone balance and reduce inflammation.

5. Avoiding Environmental Toxins: Exposure to environmental toxins, such as pesticides and chemicals, can negatively impact fertility outcomes in women with endometriosis.

Avoiding exposure to these toxins as much as possible can help improve fertility outcomes.

6. Smoking Cessation: Smoking has been linked to reduced fertility outcomes in women with endometriosis. Quitting smoking can improve overall health and fertility outcomes.

It is important to note that lifestyle modifications should be used in conjunction with medical treatments recommended by a healthcare provider. Women with endometriosis should speak with their healthcare provider before making any significant lifestyle changes.

Partner Support and Communication During Endometriosis and Fertility Treatment

Partner support and communication are important during endometriosis and fertility treatment. Here are some ways partners can provide support and improve communication:

1. Emotional Support: Endometriosis and fertility treatment can be emotionally taxing on women.

Partners can provide emotional support by being empathetic and understanding of their partner's feelings. They can also offer a listening ear and provide comfort when needed.

2. Education and Advocacy: Partners can educate themselves about endometriosis and fertility treatment to better understand their partner's condition and treatment. They can also act as an advocate for their partner during medical appointments and treatment.

3. Practical Support: Partners can provide practical support, such as helping with household chores or running errands, to alleviate stress and allow their partner to rest.

4. Communication: Open and honest communication is crucial during endometriosis and fertility treatment. Partners can encourage their partners to express their feelings and concerns, and they can share their feelings and concerns as well. They can also work together to make decisions regarding treatment and other aspects of their lives.

5. Involvement: Partners can be involved in the treatment process by attending appointments and learning about treatment options. They can also participate in fertility treatments, such as IVF, by providing sperm for insemination or donating eggs.

Partners should also take care of their own physical and emotional health during endometriosis and fertility treatment. They can seek support from a therapist or counselor if needed.

CHAPTER FIVE

PREGNANCY AND BIRTH OUTCOMES IN WOMEN WITH ENDOMETRIOSIS

Endometriosis is a condition in which tissue similar to the lining of the uterus grows outside of the uterus, causing pain and discomfort. There is evidence to suggest that endometriosis may have an impact on pregnancy and birth outcomes in women.

Studies have shown that women with endometriosis may have a higher risk of pregnancy complications such as miscarriage, preterm birth, and caesarean section delivery. Endometriosis can also increase the risk of certain pregnancy-related conditions, such as gestational hypertension and preeclampsia.

Additionally, endometriosis can affect fertility and make it more difficult for women to conceive. In some cases, women with endometriosis may require fertility treatments such as in vitro fertilization (IVF) to become pregnant.

However, it's important to note that not all women with endometriosis will experience negative pregnancy and birth outcomes. With proper medical management and monitoring during pregnancy, many women with endometriosis can have healthy pregnancies and births.

If you have endometriosis and are planning to become pregnant, it's important to talk to your healthcare provider about your risks and options for managing your condition during pregnancy.

Future Directions in Endometriosis and Fertility Research and Treatment

Endometriosis is a complex condition that can have a significant impact on a woman's fertility and reproductive health. While there have been significant advances in our understanding and treatment of endometriosis, there is still much that we don't know, and there is a need for ongoing research to improve our ability to diagnose and treat the condition.

Some of the future directions in endometriosis and fertility research and treatment include:

1. Developing new diagnostic tools: Currently, the only way to definitively diagnose endometriosis is through surgery. However, researchers are working to develop less invasive diagnostic tools, such as blood tests or imaging techniques, that could help identify the condition earlier and more accurately.

2. Improving treatment options: While there are several treatments available for endometriosis, including surgery and hormonal therapies, they are not always effective or appropriate for all patients. Researchers are exploring new treatment options, such as gene therapy or immunotherapy, that could target the underlying causes of endometriosis more effectively.

3. Focusing on personalized medicine: Endometriosis is a highly individualized condition, with significant variation in symptoms, severity, and response to treatment between patients. Researchers are exploring ways to use personalized medicine approaches,

such as genetic testing or biomarker analysis, to tailor treatments to individual patients.

4. Improving fertility outcomes: For women with endometriosis who are struggling with infertility, there is a need for more effective fertility treatments that can help them conceive. Researchers are exploring new approaches, such as ovarian tissue transplantation or regenerative medicine, to improve fertility outcomes in women with endometriosis.

Overall, there is a growing recognition of the importance of endometriosis research and the need to develop more effective treatments for this condition. With ongoing research and collaboration between clinicians, researchers, and patients, we can hope to improve the lives of millions of women affected by endometriosis.

CONCLUSION

Endometriosis is a condition in which tissue similar to the lining of the uterus grows outside of the uterus, causing pain and discomfort. This condition can also have a significant impact on a woman's fertility, making it more difficult for her to conceive. However, there are several treatment options available to help manage the condition and improve fertility outcomes.

One common treatment for endometriosis and fertility concerns is laparoscopic surgery. During this procedure, the surgeon uses a small camera to look inside the pelvic cavity and remove any endometriosis tissue that is present. This can help improve fertility outcomes for women with mild to moderate endometriosis by removing any blockages or adhesions that may be interfering with conception.

In addition to surgery, hormonal therapies may also be used to manage symptoms of endometriosis and improve fertility outcomes. Birth control pills or other forms of hormonal contraception can help regulate the menstrual cycle and reduce the growth of endometrial tissue. Other hormonal treatments, such as gonadotropin-releasing hormone (GnRH) agonists, can also be used to temporarily induce a state of menopause and reduce endometriosis symptoms.

For women who are unable to conceive through natural means, fertility treatments such as in vitro fertilization (IVF) may be recommended. IVF involves fertilizing an egg outside of the body and then implanting it into the uterus.